Patrícia Yanne de Oliveira
Mariane F. L. Lacerda
Caroline F. M. Girelli

The location of the radiographic apex and apical foramen in molars

Patrícia Yanne de Oliveira
Mariane F. L. Lacerda
Caroline F. M. Girelli

The location of the radiographic apex and apical foramen in molars

ScienciaScripts

Cover image: www.ingimage.com

This book is a translation from the original published under ISBN 978-613-9-65066-8.

Publisher:
Sciencia Scripts
is a trademark of
Dodo Books Indian Ocean Ltd. and OmniScriptum S.R.L publishing group

120 High Road, East Finchley, London, N2 9ED, United Kingdom
Str. Armeneasca 28/1, office 1, Chisinau MD-2012, Republic of Moldova, Europe
Printed at: see last page
ISBN: 978-620-7-84996-3

SUMMARY

Determining the working length (WL) is of paramount importance for instrumentation, obturation and the efficiency of endodontic treatment. The radiographic method is the one most used by dental surgeons to obtain this length; and in this method, the radiographic apex is of great importance, as it is the vital reference for obtaining the WL. However, the exit of the apical foramen is the ideal anatomical landmark sought to delimit the endodontic procedure. However, these two entities do not always coincide. The aim of this study was to determine the location of the apical foramen of the distal root of mandibular first molars, comparing it with the radiographic apex. To this end, an in vitro study was carried out in which 30 mandibular first molars were selected, in which files were inserted up to the exit of the foramen and these were radiographed. These radiographs were then subjected to measurement software. Crown/radiographic apex and crown/apical foramen measurements were collected. The data was tabulated and sent for statistical analysis. The results showed statistically significant differences between the crown/radiographic apex and crown/apical foramen measurement groups, with 33.33% of the samples coinciding. In the 66.67% that did not coincide, the measurements ranged from 0.3mm to 1.20mm, with a range of 0.90, a mean of 0.71mm and a standard deviation of 0.30mm. It was observed that there is a considerable discrepancy between the location of the radiographic apex and the exit of the foramen in the distal root of mandibular first molars, which can influence the entire course of treatment of the canal system and have the immediate consequence of the failure of endodontic therapy.

Keywords: Radiographic Apex; Anatomical; Odontometry; Radiography, Distal; First Molar, Inferior, apical foramen.

SUMMARY

CHAPTER 1

INTRODUCTION

According to Pécora et al. (2004a), the anatomy of the root canal system dictates the parameters under which endodontic treatment will be carried out and affects the chances of success. The anatomy of each tooth has common characteristics as well as very complex variations. Knowledge of the anatomy of the root canals is of great help to the professional, from the access surgery to the obturation of the canals, and is a sure-fire way of achieving success and avoiding unpleasant situations.

In order to carry out endodontic therapy effectively, it is necessary to know the correct location of the apical foramen, as this anatomical landmark delimits the scope of both instrumentation and obturation (GUTMANN and LEONARD, 1995).

Gutmann and Leonard (1995) state that determining the location of the apical foramen is of paramount importance for the course and success of endodontic therapy, since it is from the precise location of the foraminal exit that the CT is obtained, in order to determine the future of endodontic treatment.

Thus, determining the CT is a fundamental condition for successful endodontic treatment, in order to avoid errors in this therapy, which can result in periapical perforations, over instrumentation, over obturation, post-operative pain, as well as poor and incomplete instrumentation and obturation (GUTMANN and LEONARD, 1995).

In order to determine where this important anatomical landmark is located and consequently obtain the CT, professionals can use various methods, such as tactile, radiographic and electronic techniques (SIU et al, 2009).

The conventional radiographic method is the most widely used (TOSUN et al., 2008). However, this method's effectiveness has been questioned in some studies, because due to the morphological variations of the root canal system, the apical foramen almost always does not correspond to the radiographic apex, and errors can occur during interpretation (ABBOT, 1987).

According to Scarparo and Neuvald (2006), well-defined data can be observed in relation to the non-coincidence of the apical foramen exit with the dental apex itself; the average values of this difference ranged from 0.38mm to 0.99mm, reaching a maximum distance of 3mm.

Thus, the importance of the precise location of the foramen exit is emphasised, as it is a preponderant factor for efficient instrumentation and correct obturation of the canal system and, consequently, a determining factor in its success.

Given this context, it is clear that it is important to carry out a study on the location of the apical foramen exit and its correlation with the radiographic apex, given that this is the conventional radiographic method most commonly used to measure the TC.

CHAPTER 2

LITERATURE REVIEW

2.1 ANATOMIES

2.1.1 External Tooth - 1st lower molar

The first permanent lower molar is generally the largest of the human teeth. They erupt between the ages of six and seven, distal to the deciduous second molars, with the root completing between the ages of nine and ten. It has a complex morphology and can almost always be pentacuspidate and biradicular, containing a mesial root and a distal root (DE DEUS, 1992).

According to Soares and Goldberg (2001), the lower first molar is the first permanent tooth to erupt in the mouth and is also the one most in need of endodontic intervention. It has a crown with five cusps, three buccal and two lingual.

The roots, with a common base, are most often distal and mesial. Both roots have longitudinal grooves, the deepest of which are on the mesial root. The distal root is often slightly shorter and straighter than the mesial root. When the lower first molar has a third root, this is the lingual one. The incidence of three roots in this tooth is low in people of Caucasian origin (5%) and high in people of Mongolian origin (20%). The third root is located in the lingual-distal position. When starting endodontic treatment on a lower first molar, all these possibilities should be borne in mind (PÉCORA et al.,

2004a).

2.1. 2The canal - 1st lower molar

Estrela and Figueiredo (1999) pointed out that knowledge of the internal dental anatomy is fundamental for the perfect execution of the root canal sanitation and modelling process. The anatomical structure of the pulp cavity is considered to be very complex, as checking its macro-configuration, illustrated by drawings, photographs, diaphanisations (decalcifications), mouldings, serial cuts (wear) and computer analysis, can often be illusory, as it does not give an approximate and projected idea of the internal micromorphology. And the variety of internal shapes present in the different dental groups cannot be underestimated, as in some situations we may come across quite atypical anatomical features, and it is necessary to know how to identify them so as not to increase the risk of errors in root canal treatment.

Soares and Goldberg (2001) say that when the lower first molar has three canals, the distal one is wide, approximately oval in shape (with a long axis in the buccal-lingual direction) and gently curved or sometimes straight. When there are four canals, the distal two are smaller than in the case of a single canal. When there are two canals, they are generally wide and oval-shaped, arranged in a vestibulo-lingual direction, following the root anatomy. The incidence of lower molars with four canals in their studies is 36 per cent, although some researchers differ on these findings. Other authors say that the differences lie in the criteria for classifying one category or another and this leads to a variability of results.

In addition to these variations, Pécora et al. (2004a) explained that these teeth can have three roots and all the variations mentioned above. In this way, it is possible to see the enormous anatomical variation that can be present in the lower first molar. The root canals of the lower first molar open at the mesial and distal edges of the pulp chamber floor and vary greatly in number and shape. Although in most cases lower first molars have two roots, the number of root canals can vary as follows:

a) two canals in the mesial root and one canal in the distal root;

b) two canals in the mesial root and two canals in the distal root;

c) three canals in the mesial root and one in the distal root;

d) three canals in the mesial root and two canals in the distal root.

Carvalho et al. (2007) emphasised the importance of knowing the root anatomical variations in mandibular molars, especially the presence of an additional canal in the distal position. They reported a clinical case of a lower molar with two roots and four root canals, describing the operative sequence applied. They noted that knowledge of dental anatomy and morphology is extremely important for correct endodontic treatment. In this study, the lower first molar had two roots (mesial and distal) and four root canals, two mesial and two distal. The difficulties encountered throughout the treatment involved opening the pulp chamber, localising the canals, instrumentation and filling. We therefore suggest the use of good lighting, careful examination of the floor with exploratory files, X-rays in case of doubt and, if possible, visual magnification, using available resources, in order to locate a possible fourth canal.

According to Pérez et al. (2012), the internal anatomy of the tooth imposes limitations on the correct preparation of the root canal, due to its numerous variations such as irregularities, isthmuses, ramifications, presence of curvatures, among others, which can often jeopardise the main objective of endodontic therapy.

2.1.3 From the Apical Foramen

Kuttler (1955) studied the root apices of extracted human teeth using light microscopy. The aim of this study was to analyse the topography and anatomy of the root apex, as well as the direction, shape, diameter and location of the foramen, in addition to the size and thickness of the apical cementum. He found that the older the individual, the greater the thickness of the apical cementum, shifting the foramen away from the apical apex. The author emphasised that the root apex and the final portion of the tooth root occupy approximately 1/3 of its length. As characteristics, he also noted that the terminal portion of the root apex is called the apical vertex, and that the apical foramen is the circumference that separates the end of the canal from the external surface of the root. He also analysed that the root canal in the occlusal-apical direction is made up of two conical-truncated canals, which are juxtaposed by their apexes. Finally, he observed that the dentinal canal has its walls lined with dentin, which converge towards the end of the root, up to a maximum constriction.

Hess, Culieras and Lamiable (1983) elucidated that the union of the apically converging dentin canal with the apically diverging cementum canal constitutes the most important anatomical reference point in endodontics: the so-called cemento-dentin-canal boundary or CDC boundary. The authors found that most of the time, the main root canal does not open apically in a single shape, but in accessory and secondary canals which, forming the apical delta, open into smaller foramina with diameters of between 60 and 80 micrometres.

According to Pécora et al. (2004b), the end of the root canal (apical foramen) is almost always located on one side of the root and very rarely at its apex, even in straight roots, with the foramen located para-apically. The mouth of the canal in the vicinity of the apex rarely coincides rectilinearly, usually on one side of the root. The apical foramen is distant from the root apex, and this distance can vary from 0.5 to 3.0mm laterally from the root, more frequently distally: D - 48%. C- centre of the apex.

Figure 1 shows the anatomical points in the apical third of greatest interest (RAMOS and BRAMANTE, 2005):

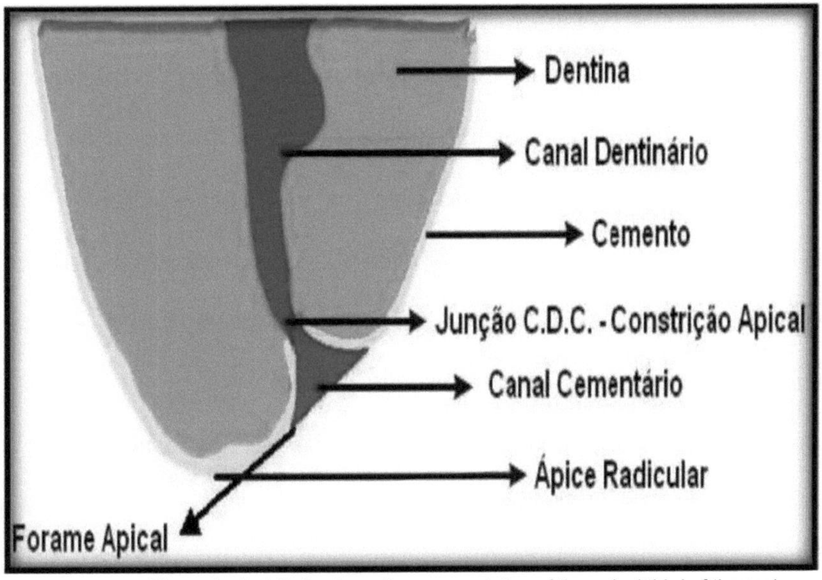

Figure 1 - Detailed schematic representation of the apical third of the root.
Source: (RAMOS and BRAMANTE, 2005, p. 5).

a) Root apex: corresponds to the extreme limit of the root;

b) Apical foramen (AF): this is the region of the root canal bounded by the cementum tissue, which lines the external portion of the dentin, and the place where the vascular-nervous bundle penetrates from the periapical region into the pulp cavity;

c) Cemento-dentin-canal junction (CDC): this is the junction between the dentin canal and the cementum canal, and is usually the point where the root canal has the smallest diameter. It can vary in shape and position, or even be absent. Also known as apical constriction (AC);

d) Dentinal canal: walls lined with dentin, which converge towards the end of the root.

e) Cementary canal: divergent walls lined with cementum that open onto the outer wall of the root (VELHO, 2011).

Nekoofar et al. (2006) found that the root canal is basically made up of two main conical sections. One formed by a cone of dentin with the base facing the coronal part of the tooth, and a cone formed by cementum with the base facing the apex of the tooth. This results in the shape of two inverted cones connected by their apexes, similar to an hourglass called a CDC. At or near the meeting point of these two cones is the smallest diameter of the root canal. This constriction is located approximately 0.5mm from the apical foramen and has a diameter of approximately 0.22mm.

According to Wrbas et al. (2007), the site with the smallest canal diameter is where the change from pulp tissue to periodontal tissue takes place, and as such is the site of choice to serve as the limit in cases of endodontic therapy. As it is a purely histological point, this location is unfeasible in the endodontic clinic, as in order to determine it correctly it would be necessary to extract the tooth and make histological sections to locate this point (SIU et al., 2009).

Apical constriction is often described as the point at which root canal obturation should extend and according to Peres et al. (2010) the obturation limit could affect the success of endodontic treatment, although the prognosis is worse when there is significant over- or under-obturation. Also according to Peres et al. (2010), the apical third presents the greatest anatomical complications, such as curvatures and atresias, and the variable position of the main foramen in relation to the root apex is also emphasised.

According to Zani et al. (2010), most root canals do not end in a rounded apex with an opening, and 75% of root canals in the apical third are actually irregular or oval in shape.

Burgel and Borba (2011) used scanning electron microscopy (SEM) to determine the average diameter of the main foramen of the root canal of mandibular premolars, the distance between the main foramen and the apex of the root canal, and to determine the location of the main foramen. They concluded that in only 9.1% of cases did the main foramen end exactly at the apical vertex, with the average distance to this point in mandibular premolars being 1.1mm for the first and 1.0mm for the second premolars.

According to Bath-Balogh and Fehrenbach (2012), the apical foramen is the opening at the apex of the tooth through which the pulp communicates with the surrounding periodontal ligaments. If there is more than one foramen in a root, the widest is called the apical foramen and the others are accessory foramens. This opening is surrounded by layers of cementum and allows structures such as arteries, veins and nerves to enter and exit. Thus, communication between the pulp and the periodontal ligaments is possible via the apical foramen. The apical foramen is the last part of the tooth to form; this occurs after the crown has erupted into the oral cavity. In the developing tooth, the foramen is wide and located in the centre. However, as the tooth matures, its diameter decreases and it is displaced from its position. The foramen may be located at the apex of the root, but it is usually slightly displaced in an occlusal direction.

2.2 ODONTOMETRY

2.2.1 Radiographic odontometry and the radiographic apex

The inaccuracy of the conventional radiographic method can lead to errors in calculating the CT, which result in over- or under-instrumentation and, consequently, inadequate fillings (PALMER et al., 1971).

Bramante and Berbert (2002) indicated the use of radiographic techniques, with variations in the vertical and horizontal angle, to aid diagnosis and observe the anatomy of root canals, such as the Clark and triangular tracing techniques.

Friedman (2002) reported that obtaining the CT based on radiographic interpretation has been the method most used by clinicians and specialists in endodontic therapy, more precisely in determining the CT. This has provided satisfactory results, despite the technical limitations of this method. The author emphasised that radiographs have long been used as the main measure to assess the outcome of endodontic therapy. However, radiographs are subject to changes due to angulation and contrast, as well as the interpretation of examiners. Due to these inconsistent and biased interpretations, radiographs can compromise the reliability of the results.

According to Pécora et al. (2004b), radiographs of the tooth can reveal a large part of the internal anatomy which, combined with theoretical knowledge, dictates the size of the drill to be used in the access surgery, its direction, the size of the first instrument to be used inside the root canal and also which modifications should be used to prepare the endodontic cavity in order to facilitate localisation of the root canals.In order to know the exact CT value, it is necessary to establish two points: the external reference and the apical limit that will determine the end point of the instrumentation. By determining these two points, we obtain the CT.

Omer et al. (2004) compared the diaphanisation technique with radiography in visualising the anatomy of the root canals of maxillary first molars. The authors analysed, among other things, the position and number of apical foramina. In conclusion, the study demonstrated the limited value of the radiographic technique in analysing these anatomical aspects.

According to Scarfe et al. (2006), radiographic examination is an essential component in understanding and managing endodontic problems. It is therefore fundamental in all aspects, such as diagnosis and endodontic treatment planning.

Baldi (2005) explained that methods that use radiographic image interpretations have limitations resulting from factors such as distortions, impossibility of visualising the apical foramen and constriction, anatomical interferences and clinical instruments, such as clamps, used during endodontic treatment. There is also the restriction of being a two-dimensional image of a three-dimensional object, as well as the subjective interpretation of the operator.

According to Scarfe et al. (2006), the amount of information obtained from conventional radiographs is limited by the fact that the three-dimensional anatomy is being compressed into a two-dimensional image. As a result of this superimposition of images, the radiograph reveals limited aspects of the three-dimensional anatomy.

According to Zani et al. (2010), the diameter and dimension of oval canals cannot be detected radiographically and preparations made by endodontic files do not allow access along the dimension, leaving instrumentation and obturation incomplete, thus serving as a possible source of future endodontic failure.

According to Peres et al. (2010), although it is the routinely used and, until now, irreplaceable resource in the endodontic clinic, periapical radiographic examination provides an inaccurate position of the endodontic instrument in relation to the foramen. The authors compared the discrepancy between the conventional odontometry method and the standard reference determined visually. They concluded that only 50.5% of the roots had visual odontometry that coincided with radiographic odontometry. Premolars were the group with the greatest discrepancy, followed by molars and anterior teeth.

Valverde (2011) pointed out that in traditional odontometry, which is widely used and is carried out using radiographic images, the radiographic tooth apex is considered the reference for establishing the length of the tooth and, consequently, the TC. The author also explained that the problems with the radiographic method occur during the radiographic measurements and their interpretation. These problems occur due to the following facts: radiography is the two-dimensional projection of a three-dimensional object, which leads to superimposition and distortion of images, morphological variations in the root canal system; the apical foramen does not always correspond to the radiographic apex; there are errors during the observer's radiographic interpretation; the time spent taking and processing radiographs; and the potential risk to the health of the patient and professional.

According to Leonardo and Leonardo (2012), morphologically there is a great variety in the distance between the radiographic apex and the exit of the apical foramen, demonstrating that branching in the apical area is the rule, not the exception. The actual location of the apical foramen is clinically impossible to ascertain until the root canal has been completely filled. The radiographic method for determining the apical limit does not take anatomical variables into account. This often leads, in cases of live pulp, to over-instrumentation, traumatic injury to the apical periodontal tissue and consequent post-operative pain. Clinically, this is one of the reasons why the operator, even at the beginning of endodontic treatment, feels uncertain about detecting the position of the foraminal exit and establishing the CRT.

2.2.2 Electronic odontometry

Ferreira et al. (1998) clinically analysed the effectiveness of two auxiliary methods in odontometry: the millimetre screen and the electronic apex locator (APIT, Osada, Japan). The results were concordant in 76.47 per cent of cases when it came to teeth with vital pulp, and in teeth with necrotic pulp the results were concordant in 83.64 per cent of cases. APIT was not efficient in determining root length only in obliterated canals or those with apexes that showed major resorption. The millimetre mesh was less effective in determining root length due to its own radiographic limitations. The electronic locator proved to be more efficient than the millimetre screen, but it is expensive.

Ferreira (2000) compared the effectiveness of three methods: the conventional radiographic method (KODAK Ektaspeed Plus film), the digital radiographic method (DenOptix) and the electronic method (Apit apical Iocaliser) in determining the CT for endodontics in human teeth in vitro. The results showed that there was no statistically significant difference between the three odontometry methods investigated for the three groups of teeth. The electronic method, Apit, had an average accuracy rate of 88.9%, while the conventional radiographic method and the digital method had an accuracy rate of 95.5%. All three odontometry methods had a high accuracy rate and were therefore considered reliable.Baldi (2005) assessed the influence of foramen diameter and endodontic instrument on the odontometric reading of two electronic apex locators (Root ZX® and NovApex®). Teeth with a smaller diameter foramen showed a more accurate measurement with the apex locator than teeth with a larger diameter foramen, which showed a greater discrepancy in the measurement. The use of No. 10 K files on teeth with larger foramen diameters was more accurate when compared to files that coincided with the foramen diameters for the Root ZX® appliance. For the NovApex®, this correlation only started to occur after file no. 40.

Real (2006), in an "in *vitro*" study, compared the effectiveness of odontometry obtained using the Elements Diagnostic, Root Zx and Just II electronic apical locators, with canals irrigated with 1% sodium hypochlorite and also with canals irrigated with 0.9% saline solution, at different times. It was concluded that there was a statistically significant difference at the 5% level in three situations between the mean measurements obtained using the electronic apical locators and the gold standard measurements and in four situations when comparing the mean measurements obtained using the electronic apical locators and the mean measurements obtained using direct digital radiography. All the electronic methods used in this study showed low accuracy when compared to the gold standard, but with a safety percentage of 89% to 95% in positioning the files within the limits of the root canals. It was also concluded in this study that the greatest certainty in positioning the files within the limits of the root canals using the electronic apical locators occurred when they were irrigated with 1% sodium hypochlorite.

Scarparo and Neuvald (2006) compared, in vivo, the TC determined by the radiographic and electronic methods in clinical situations of pulp necrosis with and without radiographically visible periapical lesions. Considering a tolerance interval of 0.5mm, there was an 80% coincidence in the measurements of the two methods, and the average difference observed was 0.33mm. Thus, there were no statistically significant differences between the measurements determined by the Ingle technique and Root ZX® ($p = 0.35$).

Bonetti et al. (2007) checked whether the CRT measurements taken by the Root ZX II apex locator were compatible with those obtained by conventional radiography and whether the electronic method could be used safely. For this study, 20 multi-rooted teeth were used in vivo, totalling 52 canals. The results showed no statistically significant differences ($p>0.05$) for both the bio and necropulpectomy cases. It was concluded that the measurements were similar for both methods and that the Root Zx II can be used safely for odontometry.

Giusti et al. (2007) assessed in vivo the reliability of the Bingo 1020 apex locator (Rishom-Lezion, Israel) in obtaining the longitudinal length of the root canal.

Electronic odontometry with the Bingo apex locator was carried out on thirty single-rooted teeth and compared with conventional odontometry associated with direct digital radiography (RVG TROPHY, Vincennes, France). The results showed the efficiency of this apex locator, as 96.67% of the measurements confirmed by direct digital radiography allowed the radiographic halo to be visualised. It was observed that the measurements obtained by the direct digital radiography system, when they did not coincide, were very close to the measurements provided by the locator. They therefore concluded that the Bingo 1020 and RVG TROPHY are reliable resources for obtaining CT scans.

Wrbas et al. (2007) carried out a study comparing the accuracy of two foraminal locators: Root ZX® and Raypex®. Single-rooted teeth with a prior indication for extraction were selected and given an initial cervical preparation using 1% NaOCl as the irrigating solution. The results showed that electronic odontometry with Root ZX® was accurate in 75% of cases and Raypex® was accurate in 80% of cases. The authors concluded that the foraminal locators tested were fairly accurate in determining root canal length.

Pascon et al. (2009) compared the accuracy of two electronic foraminal locators in vivo using a digital radiographic imaging system. The CT of 831 root canals was determined electronically using the Dentaport ZX® and Raypex 5® electronic foraminal locators and confirmed radiographically. Positive or negative values were recorded when the file tip was detected beyond or below the radiographic apex, respectively. Statistically, the two electronic foraminal locators showed no differences in accuracy within the limitations of this in vivo study.

In an in vitro study, Velho (2011) evaluated and compared the accuracy of two methods of obtaining the TC - conventional radiographic and electronic methods, comparing the measurements obtained by these with the CTR measurements of each tooth. The results obtained showed statistically significant differences ($p<0.05$) in both methods (radiographic and electronic) used at 0.5mm below the apical foramen, when compared to the CTR. The electronic method obtained results that were closer to the real thing, showing 73.3 per cent accuracy for a range of 0.5-1mm below the apical foramen.

Silva (2012) compared the accuracy of the ZX II, ZX Mini and RA A-15 electronic apex locators in localising the AF. The results showed that the average difference between these values was 0.50 mm for the ZX II, 0.45 mm for the ZX Mini and 0.50 mm for the RA A-15. With a tolerance of 0.5mm, the LAE accuracy values were 62.5%, 56.2% and 50% respectively. For a tolerance of 1.0mm, the values were 87.5%, 96.87% and 87.5%, respectively. It was concluded that the LAEs tested did not differ in terms of their accuracy in detecting AF, with the three devices pointing an average of 0.49mm below this point.

Paludo et al. (2012) evaluated, in vivo, the clinical applicability of two LAEs - Apex (Septodont) and iPex (NSK) - on different groups of human teeth using radiographic analysis. There was no statistically significant difference between Apex and iPex in terms of the measurements considered acceptable and not acceptable ($p>0.05$) or the distance between the file tip and the radiographic apex ($p>0.05$). The Apex and iPex apical locators provided reliable odontometric measurements for endodontic treatment.

According to Freitas et al. (2012), electronic foraminal locators are instruments that fulfil the role for which they were developed, i.e. they really can determine the CT work in endodontics. However, knowledge of the principle of action of each device is necessary for better use by dental professionals. Electronic foraminal locators are reliable and precise; however, despite these characteristics, they do not fulfil the need for radiographic measurements, and a combination of radiographic and electronic techniques is the best way to determine the CT.

Pereira et al. (2014) assessed the ability of the Quill® foraminal locator to determine the CT based on the location of the AF, established in this study at 1mm below the apical foramen, in a sample of 24 canals. The distance from the tip of the file to the apical foramen was measured on the SEM. The mean measurement was 1.089mm (±0.437mm). The two-tailed t-test showed that there were no significant differences (p=0.338) between the experimental values and a hypothetical tested value of 1mm. The Quill® foraminal locator was able to determine a satisfactory CT for endodontic treatment, set at 1mm below the foramen.

CHAPTER 3

OBJECTIVES

3.1 GENERAL OBJECTIVE

The aim of this study was to assess in vitro the actual location of the apical foramen of the distal root of permanent mandibular first molars.

3.2 SPECIFIC OBJECTIVES

a) To identify the difference between the location of the radiographic apex and the apical foramen in the distal root of mandibular molars;

b) Evaluate the distance, in millimetres, between the apical foramen and the radiographic apex.

CHAPTER 4

METHODOLOGY

4.1 APPROACH AND STUDY MODEL

This is an observational, descriptive, cross-sectional cohort study. The cross-sectional study model is appropriate for describing the characteristics of populations with regard to certain variables and their distribution patterns, as well as analysing their incidence and inter-relationship at a given time (SAMPIERI; COLLADO; LUCIO, 2006).

A quantitative approach was adopted in this research. Quantitative research is a method aimed at finding the magnitude and causes of social phenomena, with no interest in the subjective dimension. They are described as objective, reproducible and generalisable studies and are widely used to evaluate programmes that have a stable and measurable end product (SERAPIONI, 2000).

4.2 THE STUDY UNIVERSE

The study population consisted of permanent mandibular first molars, which are usually the largest human teeth. They are pentacuspidate and have an enlarged pulp chamber in the vestibulo-lingual direction. They have 2 roots and 3 conduits in 60% of cases, with the distal root having 1 conduit in 60% and 2 conduits in 40%, according to studies by Hess (1925), Pineda and Kuttler (1972) and De Deus (1986).

4.3 STUDY SAMPLE

This study used the distal roots of 30 human lower molars, previously sterilised in an autoclave and conditioned in sodium hypochlorite, extracted for different reasons (orthodontic, prosthetic, periodontal, among others). These teeth were in a good state of preservation and were donated by professionals in the field under terms of consent.

The distal root was chosen because it had a large variation in the canal path in its apical portion.

4.4 INCLUSION/EXCLUSION CRITERIA

The inclusion criteria were mandibular first molars with fully formed root apexes and only one foramen. Teeth with torn roots, obliterated root canals or resorption, fractures, fractured instruments or more than one foramen were excluded.

4.5 PILOT STUDY

A pilot study was carried out on three mandibular molars in order to verify the best way to achieve the most consistent results, observing the inclusion and exclusion criteria. However, the data obtained was not taken into account for the main study.

Marconi and Lakatos (2007) attribute the importance of carrying out a pilot study to the fact that it can establish the reliability, validity and operability of the data obtained, as well as providing an estimate of future results.

4.6 ETHICAL ASPECTS

This research was submitted to the Research Ethics Committee of the Vale do Rio Doce University (UNIVALE), which reported that it did not need to be assessed as it was not a research project involving living beings.

4.7 DATA COLLECTION

4.7.1 Tooth selection and preparation

Human lower first molars were autoclaved (Fig. 2) and conditioned in sodium hypochlorite.

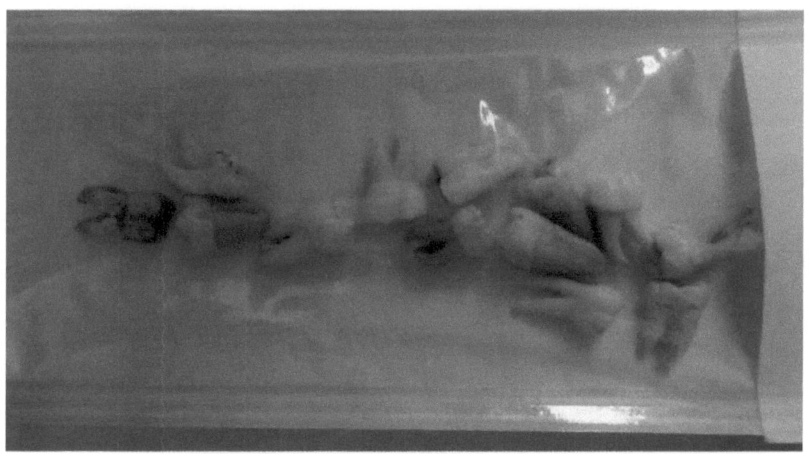

Figure 2 - Autoclaved human lower molars. Source: Experiment

The teeth were accessed coronally (Fig. 3), using cylindrical carbide drills #1557 (SS White dental articles, Rio de Janeiro, Brazil) moved at high speed, cooled by air/water, and then replaced by the Endo-Z inactive-tip truncated-conical cutter (Dentsply- Malleifer, Ballaigues, Switzerland) to carry out compensatory wear and finish the surrounding walls in order to facilitate the insertion of the file.

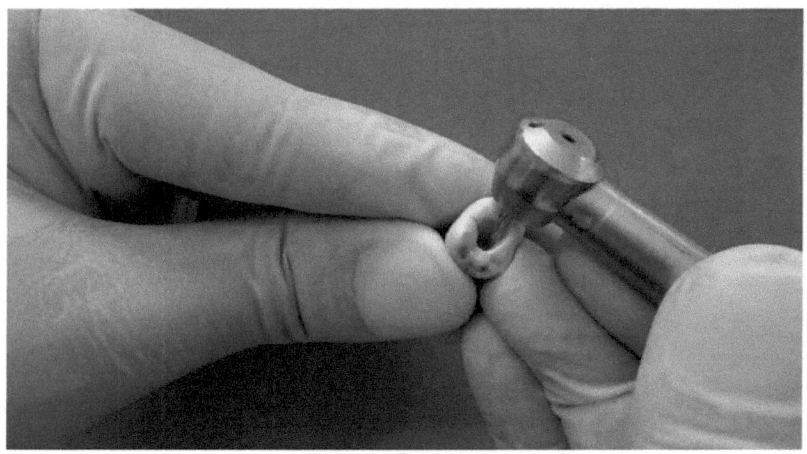

Figure 3 - Coronal access to the teeth.
Source: Experimento

After access, the teeth were numbered for control purposes (Fig. 4).

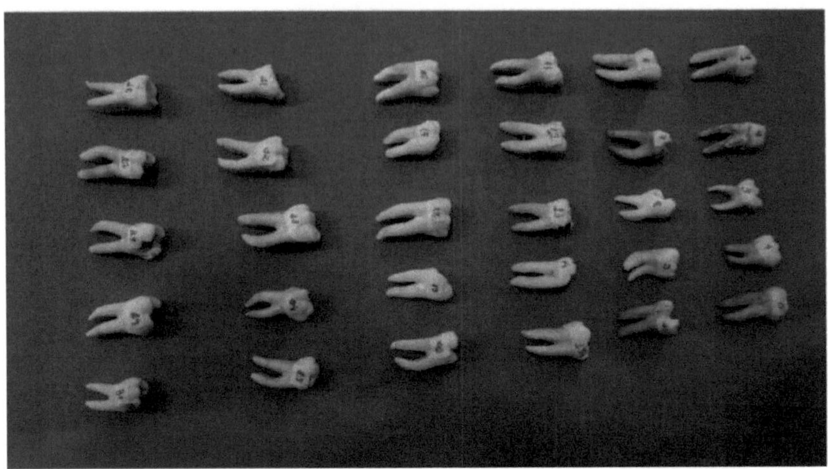

Figure 4 - Numbered lower molars for control. Source: Experiment.

The file (Fig. 5) most compatible with the diameter of the foramen was then inserted as passively as possible so as not to create any interference in the apical foramen.

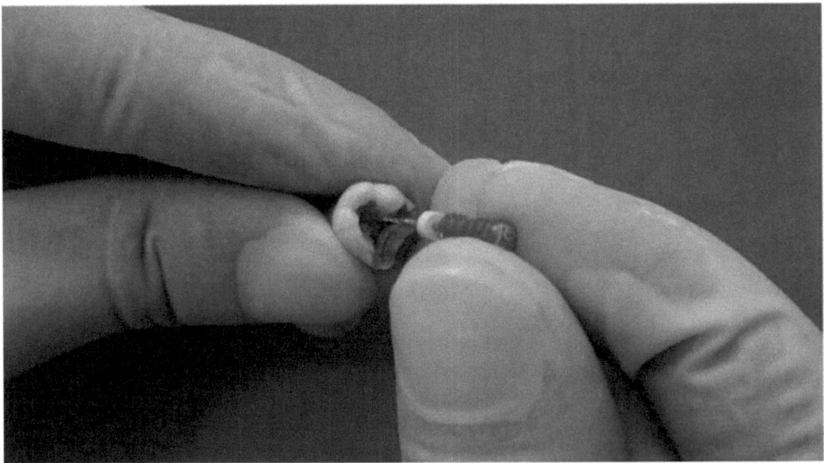

Figure 5 - File insertion. Source: Experiment

Insertion was carried out until the tip was visible, then it was retracted until it was tangent to the apical foramen (Fig. 6).

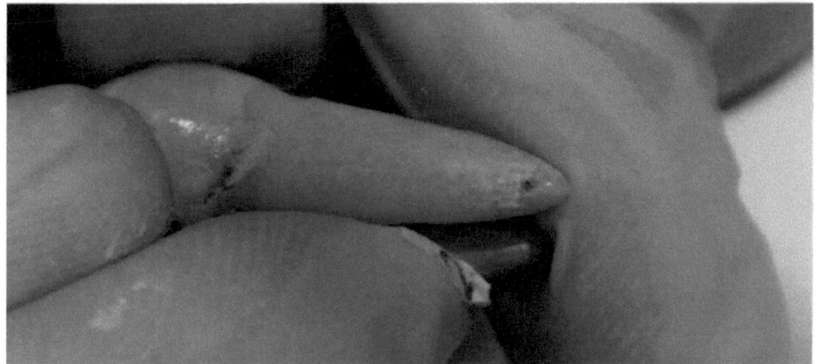

Figure 6 - Inserting the file until its tip becomes visible. Source: Experiment.

4.7.2Taking radiographs of the teeth

The tooth was then subjected to a standardised X-ray, using an angle of 90 degrees, an exposure time of 0.5 seconds and a distance of 5cm between the film and the tip of the cone (Fig. 7).

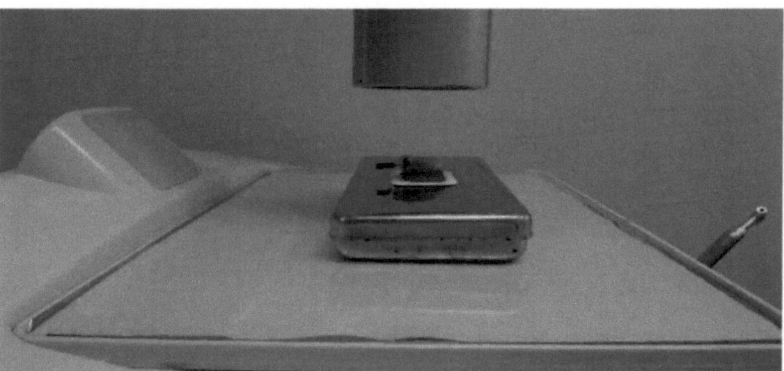

Figure 7 - Radiographic view of the tooth.
Source: Experimento

And this radiograph was also numbered to correlate it with its respective tooth (Fig. 8).

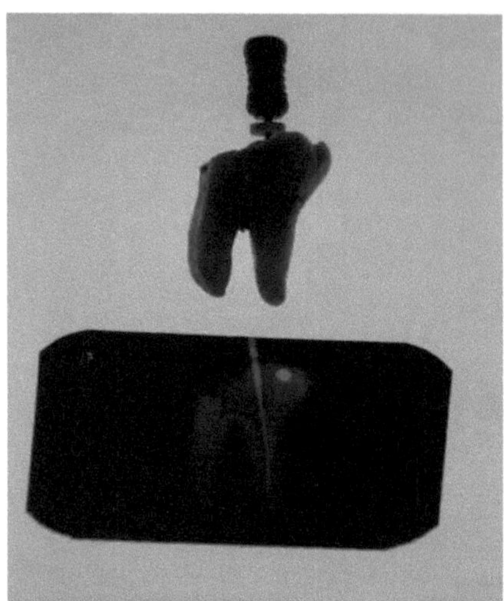

Figure 8 - Numbered tooth and X-ray. Source: Experiment.

4.7.3 Radiographic analysis and determination of Crown/Radicular Apex and Crown/Apical Foramen measurements

Radiographic analysis was then carried out and the Crown/Root Apex and Crown/Apical Foramen measurements were determined/obtained using the Radiocef Studio 2 software, which is a cephalometric tracing programme from the Radiomemory® software company (Fig. 9).

These measurements were obtained by positioning the programme's ruler on the coronal portion of the radiographic image of the tooth, extending it to the most apical portion of the radiographic image of the tooth (Crown/Root Apex Measurement) (Fig. 10). Subsequently, the Crown/Apical Foramen measurement was taken (Fig. 11), keeping the ruler positioned in the coronal portion and only repositioning its apical part over the furthest point of the file inside the canal.

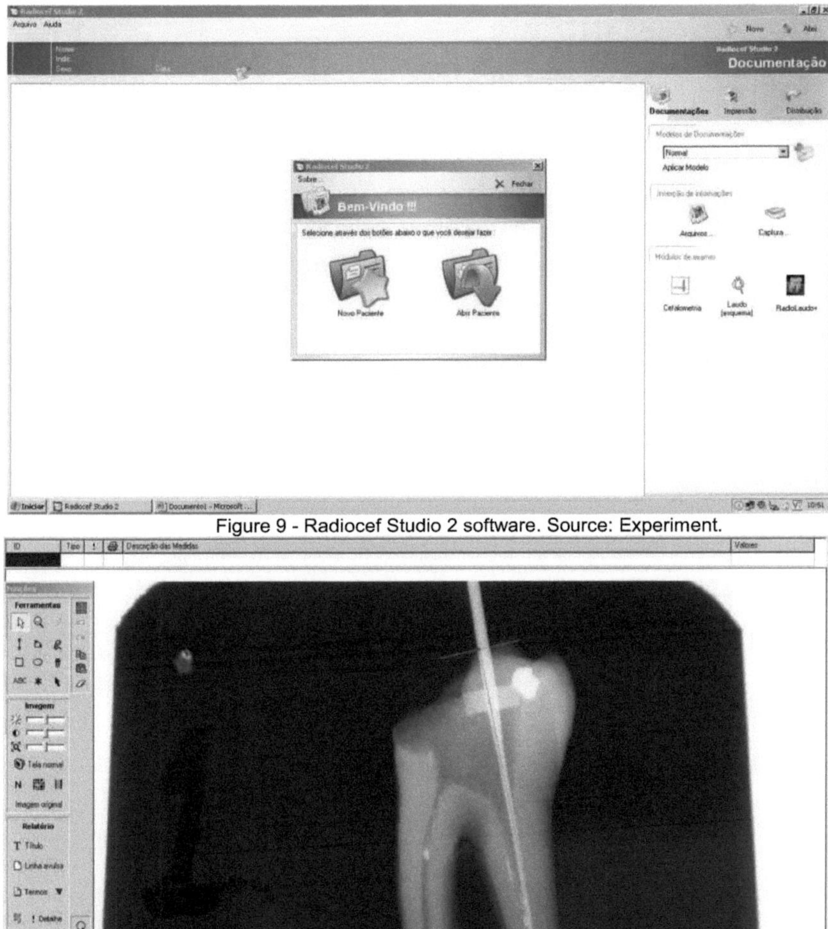

Figure 9 - Radiocef Studio 2 software. Source: Experiment.

Figure 10 - Crown/root apex measurement. Source: Experiment.

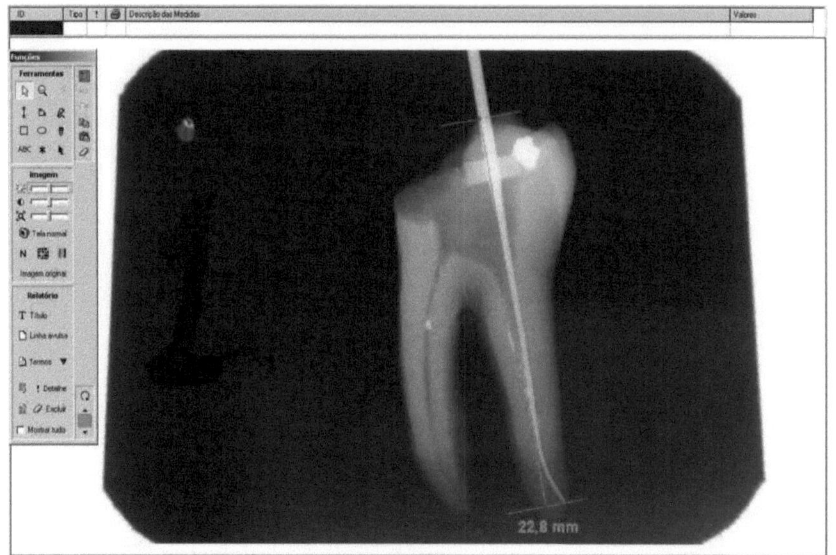

Figure 10 - Crown/Apical foramen measurement. Source: Experiment

4.7. 4Materials/instruments used

-Spherical Diamond Drill 1014 HL (KG Sorensen, Barueri, Brazil);

-Spherical Diamond Drill 1012 HL (KG Sorensen, Barueri, Brazil);

-Broca Carbide 1557 (KG Sorensen, Barueri, Brazil);

-FG 152EZ drill (KG Sorensen, Barueri, Brazil);

-Gaze Cremer (Blumenal, Brazil);

-Physiological Solution 100ml (Formas, Divinópolis, Brazil);

-Disposable 10ml syringe with needle (BD Plastipak, Curitiba, Brazil);

-Manual Limes , type K-Flexofile n 10, 25mm (Maillefer, Ballaigues, Switzerland) (6 units);

-Manual Limes , type K-Flexofile 1ª SERIE, 25mm (Maillefer, Ballaigues, Switzerland) (6 units);

-Kodak E-Speed Periapical Radiographic Film (Carestream Health, Inc.,

Rochester, USA);

-Kodak Developer (Carestream Health, Inc., Rochester, USA);

-Kodak Fixer (Carestream Health, Inc., Rochester, USA);

-Collars (Jon);

-Régua (Bandeirantes, São Paulo, Brazil);

-Adjustable clamp;

-Aspiration cannulas (Ângelus, Brazil);

-Utility Wax (Classic);

-Silicone stop (Ângelus, Brazil).

-Radiocef Studio 2 software

-Statistical

4.8 ANALYSING THE DATA

The data obtained from the measurement in the Radiocef Studio 2 programme was tabulated (Tables 1 and 2) and subjected to statistical analysis.

Table 1 - Results of the measurement of the crown at the radiographic apex (mm) and the measurement of the crown at the foramen exit (mm) and the difference between them.

TOOTH	CROWN/APICE	CROWN/FOREMAN	DIFFERENCE(mm)
1	23.60	22.60	1,00
2	21,60	21,30	0,30
3	15,70	14,70	1,00
4	1680	16,40	0,40
5	23.00	2210	0,90
6	20,20	19,10	1,10
7	20,00	19,10	0,90
8	17,20	16,70	0,50
9	17,30	17,30	0,00

10	1690	16,60	0,30
11	24,80	24,80	0,00
12	22,80	21,70	1,10
13	24,00	24,00	0,00
14	23.30	23,10	0,70
15	19.40	19,10	0,30
16	26,40	25,70	0,70
17	18,70	18,70	0,00
18	25,20	24,80	0,40
19	23,90	23,00	0,90
20	21,50	21,50	0,00
21	24.70	24,10	0,60
22	25,10	23.90	1,20
23	23.20	22, aõ	0,60
24	23.20	23.20	0,00
25	18.10	17,20	0,90
20	21,90	21,90	0,00
27	21,10	21,10	0,00
28	21,60	21,60	0,00
29	23.20	23,20	0,00
30	21,70	21,30	0,40

Table 2 - Representation of the number of samples for each difference obtained and their respective percentages.

Quantity of samples	Difference	%
10	0.00mm	33,33
3	0.30mm	10
3	On40rTim	10
1	0.50mm	3,33
2	0.6Grnm	6,66
	O.yOmm	6,66
4	0.90mm	13,2
£	1,-OOmm	6,66
2	1.10mm	666
1	1.20mm	3,33

CHAPTER 5

RESULTS

The data was analysed using descriptive and inferential statistics. SPSS software, version 19.0, was used for statistical analysis.

Quantitative variables were described using mean, standard deviation, minimum, maximum, range and quartiles. Qualitative variables were described using absolute and relative frequencies.

The paired t-test was used to compare the group means. The significance level adopted was 5%, i.e. p<0.05 was considered significant.

Table 3 - Data on the differences (mm) obtained between the crown-apex and crown-foramen measurements.

Crown - Apex	Crown - foramen	p-value
$\bar{x} \pm S$	$\bar{x} \pm S$	
21,55 ± 2,91	21,08 ± 2,92	0,000*

Paired t-test *p^0.05

There was a statistically significant difference between the crown-apex and crown-foramen measurements.

Table 4 - Data on the differences (mm) obtained from the measurements crown to radiographic apex and crown to foramen exit.

Difference (mm) between measurements Crown to radiographic apex and crown to foramen exit						
$\bar{x} \pm S$	Minimu	Maximu	Amplitude	Quartile 1	Quartile	Quartile 3

	m	m		2		
0,71 ± 0,3	0,3	1,2	0,9	0,	40,7	0,98

* The symbols $\bar{x} \pm s$ stand for mean and standard deviation respectively Range: difference between maximum and minimum.

a) Quartile 1 : 25% of the sample is below 0.40mm.

b) Quartile 2 : 50% of the sample is below 0.70mm.

c) Quartile 3 : 75% of the sample is below 0.98mm.

We observed the incidence of radiographic crown/apex measurements and crown/apical foramen in 33.33 per cent of the samples (Graph 1).

The 66.67% that didn't match ranged from 0.3mm to 1.20mm, amplitude of 0.90mm, with a mean of 0.71mm and a standard deviation of 0.30mm.

CHAPTER 6

DISCUSSION

The aim of this paper was to study the location of the apical foramen in comparison with the location of the radiographic apex on the distal root of mandibular molars, as well as to demonstrate their distance in millimetres when they do not coincide.

Lower molars were used in this study due to the higher incidence of indications for endodontic treatment and the ease with which these elements could be obtained. The distal root of the lower first molar was chosen due to the great anatomical variation in its path in the apical region and the consequent need for knowledge of internal anatomy required to avoid unsatisfactory results in endodontic treatments. This choice is in line with the study by Carvalho et al. (2007) who emphasised the importance of knowing the anatomical variations of root canals in mandibular molars, especially the presence of an additional canal in the distal position. Like Estrela and Figueiredo (1999), who state that it is important to know the internal anatomy, as its anatomical structure is very complex. Pérez et al. (2000), Soares and Goldberg (2001) and Pécora et al. (2004a) also stated that in order to carry out the root canal sanitation and modelling process perfectly, it is important to identify the internal anatomical variations so as not to increase the risk of root canal treatment errors.

After following the inclusion and exclusion criteria, 30 teeth were used in this study, totalling 30 root canals. Unlike Bonetti et al. (2007), who used 20 multi-rooted elements, or Pascon et al.

(2009), who based their research on 831 root canals and Pereira et al. (2014) who sampled 24 teeth.

In this study, the direct visual method was used to determine the exact position of the foramen, as it is the most accurate method of measuring foraminal location and it was possible to do so because the work was carried out on extracted teeth (FRIEDMAN, 2002; BALDI, 2005; REAL, 2006; BONETTI et al., 2007; CARVALHO et al., 2007; PERES et al., 2010; GRIESER, 2011).

The teeth in this study were radiographed with the file positioned in the apical foramen to visualise the location of the radiographic apex and apical foramen in a single image, as was also done in the studies by Ferreira et al. (1998), Ferreira (2000), Baldi (2005), Real (2006), Scarparo and Neuvald (2006), Bonetti et al. (2007), Wrbas et al. (2007), Pascon et al. (2009), Perez et al. (2010), Velho (2011), Leonardo and Leonardo (2012), Paludo et al. (2012), Silva (2012) and Pereira et al. (2014). However, Scarfe et al. (2006), Zani et al. (2010) and Pérez et al. (2012) used computerised tomography. The choice of radiography was due to its ease of execution and low cost.

To obtain the odontometry, two points were used, as recommended by Pécora et al. (2004), who indicated the use of an external reference and an apical limit. In this study, the external reference was a fixed point on the crown and the apical reference was the radiographic apex, as recommended by Palmer et al. (1971), Ferreira (2000), Baldi (2005), Real (2006), Scarparo and Neuvald (2006), Bonetti et al. (2007), Giusti et al. (2007) and Pascon et al. (2009), and around the apical foramen according to Wrbas et al. (2007), Paludo et al. (2012), Silva (2012), Pereira et al. (2014).

In this study, odontometries were referred to as Crown-to-Radiographic Apex and Crown-to-Apical Foramen measurements and the Radiocef Studio 2 measurement software was used to obtain them.

The results were analysed using the Paired T-Test to compare the means of the groups with a significance level of 5%, i.e. it is considered significant when it shows a value of $p<0.05$. The study found a p-value of 0.000, showing a statistically significant difference between the location of the radiographic apex and the location of the apical foramen, which is in line with the results of Leonardo and Leonardo (2012) who stated that there is a wide variety of distances between the radiographic apex and the exit of the apical foramen. As in the studies by Ferreira et al. (1998), Peres et al. (2010), Zani et al. (2010), Silva (2012) and Baldi (2005), Scarparo and Neuvald (2006) and Paludo et al. (2012).

One of the supposed explanations for the existence of this significant statistical difference in the location of the radiographic apex and the apical foramen may be due to the fact that the foramen is hardly ever located exactly at the root apex, according to studies by Bath-Balogh and Fehrenbach (2012), who explained that it can be located at the root apex, but in general it is slightly displaced in an occlusal direction. As stated by Pécora (2004a), the foramen is very rarely found at the apical apex, even in straight roots, but is located para-apically. Burgel and Borba (2011) pointed out that in only 9.1% of cases did the main foramen end exactly at the apical vertex.

The coincidence between the location of the radiographic apex and the apical foramen in this study was demonstrated in 33.33% of the samples, a result that follows in the same direction as the studies by Zani et al. (2010) who found 30% of elements that coincided. Peres et al. (2010), in their study, found a coincidence of 50.5%.

Ferreira et al. (1998) found a coincidence of 76.47% and Ferreira (2000) showed an average hit rate of 88.9%. For Giusti et al. (2007) 96.67% of the measurements were confirmed.

In 66.67% of the samples in this study, there was a difference between the location of the radiographic apex and the apical foramen. This difference averaged 0.71mm. This result is much higher than studies with significant differences, such as those by Silva (2012), who found an average of 0.49 mm. Scarparo and Neuvald (2006) found an average of 0.33 mm. Zani et al. (2010) found an average of 0.5 to 1 mm below the radiographic apex (desirable value).

The results of this study suggest that it is not possible to determine the exact location of the foramen using the radiographic method alone, as it has many shortcomings for this purpose, according to studies by Olson et al. (1991), Ferreira et al. (1998), Whaites et al. (2003), Omer et al. (2004), Baldi (2005), Peres et al. (2010), Valverde (2011) and Leonardo and Leonardo (2012), Scarfe et al. (2006) who found that radiographs have diagnostic limitations due to the fact that two-dimensional images of three-dimensional objects are obtained and images are superimposed. According to Palmer et al. (1971), these limitations can lead to inappropriate fillings. Leonardo and Leonardo (2012) emphasised the consequences of post-operative pain. However, despite these technical limitations, Clouse (1991), Friedman (2002) and Valverde (2011) emphasised that radiography provides satisfactory results, specifically in determining the CT.

Due to the large number of deficiencies present in the radiographic method for determining the apical foramen and, consequently, obtaining the TC, it is recommended that alternatives be sought through other resources available in dentistry, given the importance of this anatomical landmark in the prognosis of endodontic treatments. Apical locators are an efficient option for this function, which is also agreed upon in the studies by Ferreira et al. (1998), Paludo et al. (2012), Freitas et al. (2012), who state that electronic apical locators provide reliable odontometric measurements for endodontic treatment.

Despite the qualities presented by electronic apex locators for obtaining length compared to the radiographic method, Freitas et al. (2012) emphasised that they do not replace radiographic measurements and that a combination of radiographic and electronic techniques is therefore recommended. Scarparo and Neuvald (2006) found no significant differences between the LC determined by the radiographic and electronic methods.

Based on this study, there is a need for further research in this field, with the aim of gaining a more detailed understanding of the foraminal location of each group of teeth, in order to give dental surgeons a greater degree of knowledge so that they can carry out endodontic procedures more safely.

CHAPTER 7

CONCLUSION

There is a considerable discrepancy between the radiographic apex and the exit of the foramen in the distal root of the mandibular first molars.

The radiographic apex and apical foramen did not coincide in 66.33% of the samples, with an average difference of 0.71mm between them. There was only a correlation between the institutes in 33.67% of the cases.

These conclusions are of paramount importance because the location of the radiographic apex and apical foramen are used as a reference for obtaining the CT, a predominant factor in the success of endodontic treatment.

REFERENCES

ABBOT, P. V. Clinical Evaluation of electronic root canal measuring device. Austral. Dent. J. v. 32, n. 1, p. 17-21. 1987.

BALDI, J. V. Influence of the diameter of the apical foramen and the calibre of the endodontic instrument on the odontometric readings provided by two apical locator devices. 2005. Dissertation (Master's in Endodontics) - Bauru School of Dentistry, University of São Paulo, Bauru, 2005. Available at : <http://www.teses.usp.br/teses/disponiveis/25/25138/tde-09022007- 101948/>. Accessed on: 4 June 2015.

BATH-BALOGH, M.; FEHRENBACH, M. J. Anatomy, histology and embryology of teeth and orofacial structures. Rio de Janeiro: Elsevier, 2012.

BONETTI, C. et al. Comparative evaluation of two methods in odontometry: electronic and radiographic. Arq Bras Odontol, v. 3, n. 1, p. 17-24, 2007.

BRAMANTE, C.M.; BERBERT, A. Radiographic resources in endodontic diagnosis and treatment. 3. ed. São Paulo: Pancast, 2002.

BURGEL, M. O.; BORBA, M. G. Scanning electron microscopy analysis of the apical anatomy of mandibular premolar root canals. RFO, Passo Fundo, v. 16, n. 1, p. 49-53, jan./abr. 2011.

CARVALHO, M. G. P. et al. Lower molars with four root canals: endodontic treatment. Revista de Endodontia Pesquisa e Ensino On Line, v. 3, n. 5, p 1-6, Jan./ Jun. 2007.

DE DEUS, Q.D. Endodontics. 3.ed. Rio de Janeiro: Medsi, 1986.

ESTRELA, C; FIGUEIREDO, J.AP. Endodontics: biological and mechanical principles. São Paulo: Artes Médicas, 1999, p.819.

FERREIRA, C. M. et al. Use of two alternative techniques for localising the apical foramen in Endodontics: clinical and radiographic evaluation. Rev Odontol Univ São Paulo, v. 12, n. 3, p. 241-246, jul./set. 1998.

FERREIRA, R. Comparison of odontometry by electronic, conventional and digital radiographic methods. Master's thesis: Piracicaba, SP: State University of Campinas . Piracicaba School of Dentistry, 2000.

FREITAS, F. et al. Apical locators. Revista FAIPE, v. 2, n. 2, p. 44-63 2012.

FRIEDMAN, S. Prognosis of initial endodontic Therapy. EndodonticTopics, Oxford, v.2, n.1 p.59-88, jul. 2002.

GIUSTI, E. C. et al. Electronic and digital radiographic measurements in odontometry: in vivo analysis. RGO, Porto Alegre, v. 55, n.3, p. 239-246, jul./set. 2007

GUTMANN, J. L.; LEONARD, J. E. Problem solving in endodontic working- length determination. Compend Contin Educ Dent. v. 16, n. 3, p. 288-304. 1995.

HESS, J. C.; CULIERAS, M. J.; LAMBIABLE, N. A scanning electron microscopic investigation of principal and accessory foramina on the root surfaces of human teeth: thoughts about endodontic pathology and therapeutics. J Endod. 1983 v. 9, n. 7, p. 275-81. Jul. 1983.

HESS, W. Anatomy of the root canals of the teeth of permanent dentition. New York: Willian Wood, 1925, p.1-35.

KUTTLER. Y. Microscopic investigation of root apexes. J Am Dent Assoc. v. 50, n. 5, p. 544-52. May 1955.

LEONARDO, M. R.; LEONARDO, R. T. Root canal treatment: technological advances in minimally invasive and restorative endodontics. São Paulo: Artes Medicas. 2012.

MARCONI, M. A.; LAKATOS, E. M. Técnicas de pesquisa. 6. ed. rev. ampl. São Paulo: Atlas, 2007.

NEKOOFAR, M. H. et al. The fundamental operating principles of electronic root canal length measurement devices. Int Endod J. v. 39, n. 8, p. 595-609. Aug; 2006.

OMER, O. E. et al. A comparison between clearing and radiographic techniques in the study of the root-canal anatomy maxillary first and second molars. International Endodontic Journal, Oxford, v.37, n.5, p.291-96, May 2004.

PALMER, M. et al. Position of the apical foramen in relationto endodontic therapy. Journal of the Canadian Dental Association. v. 37, n. 8, p. 305-308, 1969.

PASCON, E. A. et al. An in vivo comparison of working length determination of two frequency-based electronic apex locators. Int Endod J. v. 42, n. 11: p. 1026-31. Nov. 2009.

PALUDO, L. et al. An in vivo radiographic evaluation of the accuracy of Apex and iPex electronic Apex locators. Braz Dent J, Ribeirão Preto, v. 23, n. 1, p. 54-58, 2012.

PÉCORA, J. D. et al. Brief review of the internal anatomy of human teeth. In: Webmaster Jesus Djalma Pécora, Ribeirão Preto School of Dentistry USP. Update 03 November 2004a. Available at: <http://www.forp.usp.br/restauradora/Anat.htm> Accessed on: 14 May 2015.

PÉCORA, J. D. et al. Apical limit of endodontic preparation. In: Webmaster Jesus Djalma Pécora, Ribeirão Preto School of Dentistry USP. Update 03 November 2004b. Available at: <http://www.forp.usp.br/restauradora/limit.htm> Accessed on: 14 May 2015.

PEREIRA, K. F. S. et al. An in vivo study of working length determination with a new apex locator. Braz Dent J, Ribeirão Preto, v. 25, n. 1, p. 17-21, Feb. 2014.

PERES, A. V. S. et al. Discrepancy between conventional odontometry method and standard reference. Rev Odontol Bras Central. v. 19, n. 49, p. 168-171. 2010.

PÉREZ, C. A. F. et al. Analysis of the anatomy of the distal root canals of mandibular molars using micro-computed tomography. Bauru School of Dentistry, University of São Paulo, 2012.

PINEDA, F., KUTTLER Y. Mesiodistal and buccolingual roentgenographic investigation of 7,275 root canals. Oral Surg Oral Med Oral Phatol. v. 33, n. 1, p. 101-10. 1972.

RADIOMEMORY. Radiocef newsletter, 2009. Available at: <http://www.radiomemory.com.br>. Accessed on: 14 May 2015.

RAMOS, C. A. S.; BRAMANTE, C. M. Odontometry: fundamentals and techniques. São Paulo: Livraria Santos, 2005.

REAL, D. J. Comparative *"in* v/in" analysis of odontometry obtained using Schick direct digital radiography and Elements diagnostic, Root ZX and Just II electronic apical locators. Master's dissertation. São Paulo: Institute of Health Sciences, 2006.

SAMPIERI, R. H.; COLLADO, C. F.; LUCIO, P. B. Metodologia de Pesquisa. 3. Ed, São Paulo: McGraw Hill, 2006.

SCARFE, W. C. et al. Clinical applications of cone-beam computed tomography in dental practice. J Can Dent Assoc. v. 72, n. 1, p. 75-80, Feb. 2006.

SERAPIONI, M. Qualitative and quantitative methods: some strategies for integration. Ciência & Saúde Coletiva, v. 5, n. 1, p. 187-192. 2000.

SILVA, T. M. In vivo comparison of the accuracy of three apical locators in detecting the apical foramen. Master's dissertation. Rio de Janeiro: Estácio de Sá University, 2012.

SIU, C. et al. An in vision comparison of the root ZX ii, the apex nrg xrf, and mini apex locator by using rotary nickel titanium files. Journal of Endodontics, v. 35, p.962-965, 2009.

SOARES, I. J; GOLDBERG, F. Endodontics: techniques and fundamentals. Porto Alegre: Artes Médicas, 2001, 376p

SCARPARO, R. K.; NEUVALD, L. R. Evaluation of electronic radiographic methods for determining the actual working length in endodontics; an *in vivo* study. RFO UPF. v. 11, n. 2, p. 50-55, 2006.

TOSUN, G. et al. Accuracy of two electronic apex locators in primary teeth with and without apical resorption: a laboratory study. International Endodontic Journal, v. 41, n. 5, p.436-441, 2008.

VALVERDE, R. F. Electronic methods for apical localisation: a literature review. Monograph (Postgraduate Endodontics). Florianópolis: ICS - FUNORTE, 2011.

VELHO, V. B. S. P. R. Comparative *in vitro* study of electronic odontometry and conventional radiography. Dissertation (Master's Degree).Porto: Fernando Pessoa University: Faculty of Health Sciences, 2011

WRBAS, K. T. et al. *In vivo* comparison of working length determination with two electronic apex locators. International Endodontics Journal, Oxford, v. 40, n. 2, p. 133-8, 2007.

ZANI, M. et al. *In vitro* analysis of the apical third of endodontically treated teeth using radiographs, computed tomography, operating microscope and photographs. Revista Brasileira de Pesquisa em Saúde, v. 12, n. 3, p. 11-16, 2010.

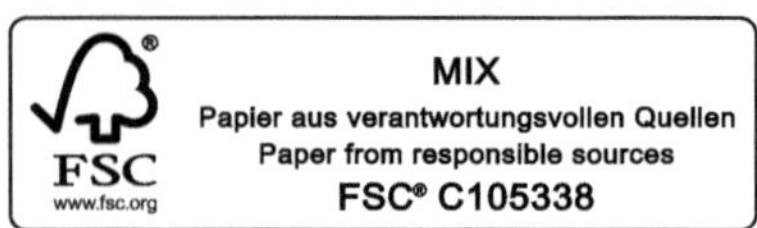

Printed by Books on Demand GmbH, Norderstedt / Germany